Nutrition,Hea
Prevention with a I

CW00430197

THE CHINA STUDY EXPLAINED

ANALYSIS Y REVIEW OF
"THE CHINA STUDY"
BY T. COLIN CAMPBELL &
THOMAS M. CAMPBELL

RUSSELL DAWSON

CONTENTS

INTRODUCTION

The China Study is a book that studies the relationship between the chronic illnesses and animal products consumption. It is considered as one of the most significant health and nutrition books ever written.

This book is based on the comprehensive nutrition study ever conducted and showed that the traditional western diet has resulted in various modern health problems and extensive growth of diseases and problems like diabetes, bowel cancer, heart disease, breast cancer, and obesity.

It is a book by T. Colin Campbell and his son Thomas M. Campbell II. They revealed that the best health with the control to reverse or stop the progress of many diseases, is the result of a plant-based diet.

The China Study was first published in January 2005, in the United States. This book concerned 65 counties in 24 different regions of China. It is an observational study, which only identifies the relationships among different variables.

According to The China Study, a particular food choice or behavior causes a certain result. It describes a massive survey of diet as well as death rates from cancer. The survey was just a monumental effort and in more than 2,400 Chinese counties to explore its implications as well as the importance of nutrition and health. As per The China Study, in the Chinese villages there are several other variables like industrialization, consumption of refined carbohydrate and sugar, exposure to chemicals, which may increase cancer risk.

The China Study gives essential, nutritional information which is life-saving for each health-seeker. Diets that eliminate entire food groups have the perspective for accidental consequences of under-consuming essential nutrients. As per the study, carrying food choices into better arrangement along with the Dietary Guidelines is a favored approach and eating more under-consumed foods like fruits, beans, low-fat dairy products, vegetables, whole grains, fish and lean meats, while also dropping the refined fats, grains, and sugars consumption is best. These changes are highly beneficial for promoting health.

The China Study uncovers unexpected answers to the most important nutritional questions of our time. The study provides the long required answers by scientists, health-conscious readers, and physicians. It answers questions like- What actually causes cancer? What will turn the epidemic of obesity? How can we extend our lives?

The China Study quickly and easily dispenses with fad diets, relying on solid and convincing evidence. In The China Study, T. Colin Campbell mentioned that, "the intake foods that contain any cholesterol more than 0 mg is unhealthy." Dr. Campbell along with his team found that proteins which are animal based, raises bad blood cholesterol levels, and on the other hand, proteins that are plant based, lowers the levels.

Result: - If one will follow The China Study, they can eventually navigate their way to tasty food that is also easy to make. Just after 6 months of eating whole or plant foods, one can see some vivid changes. The China Study findings show that with this, the person's cholesterol will drop and one can lose over 50 pounds. This also results in new hair growth.

The study cleared that the consumption of meat and dairy from hormone-injected farm animals may sensibly lift the risk of breast cancer because of increased exposure to hormones. So if we want to prevent cancer and all other diseases, then it is possible by avoiding animal protein. This will also have a great benefit to the environment as it will raise the agricultural land productivity as well as sinking the greenhouse effects of the animals.

Modern foods together with the diseases they portend, will take the dietary back seats once they are replaced by healthier ones. The China Study is an available resource that reveals potential diet-health patterns, as well as inlets for the upcoming nutritional research possibilities and prolonged awareness of the source of disease. The lessons from China make available the compelling justification for a plant-based diet to reduce the risk of diseases and promote health.

Those who want to eat bacon along with eggs for their breakfast and after that take the medication of cholesterol- lowering, should follow The China Study. However, if one want to truly take charge of your health, read it and do it soon. All those who feel some confusion concerning how to discover the healthiest path for self as well as their family, can find the finest answers in The China Study. All those looking to improve their health, performance and their success should read The China Study and follow it.

By eliminating the health harming items, one can easily live a good disease free and healthy life. The fact remains that a dietary shift on the way to Western fare unavoidably results in the creation of affluence? diseases, in spite of any changes in animal food consumption. The China Study suggests that lattice of factors or an additional factor activates this decline in health. We just have to examine the areas of convergence along with the shared lack of carbohydrates that are refined, the absence of hydrogenated oils, refined sweeteners, the weight on whole, unprocessed foods, etc. and follow the Plant diet for best results.

The study also solved the problem of some store bought foods. It cleared that store bought foods with the traditional Eskimo foods together with meat from sea and land creatures result in lower total and low-density lipoprotein cholesterol. It also results in reduced diastolic blood pressure, lowers fasting glucose, and high glucose tolerance. It shows that native diets highlighting game animals, marine mammals, berries, fish, as well as wild greens results in improved high density of lipoprotein cholesterol, and better lower triglycerides, plus, improved cardiovascular health.

So we can say that The China Study with its survey cleared most of the health and diet related problems and clarified what a person should eat and what to avoid for a healthy life and for promoting health.

CHAPTER 1.

WHAT TO LEARN FROM CHINA

China is a country that is difficult to define. It is undoubtedly on the way to attain the status of a superpower in the coming years, whereas the rest countries are struggling currently with its economic policies.

Since the late 1970s challenges, China has great achievement in western thinking regarding development as well as economic transformation in a variety of important ways. However, the development field hardly ever attempts to discover from its experience. There is no doubt in saying that China has experienced an amazing transformation in both geopolitical and economic status over the last 30 years. As the country gears its efforts to figure out the most excellent way of getting healthcare to about 1.3 billion people, the rest of the world can learn a lot from its growth and development as well as from its past successes and failures. The view of its complexity and how it got to where it is today is not captured.

China has tried numerous approaches towards development. The people of China have a strong ethical and cultural heritage, which catches priority over everything. They are uninterested to the likes of Google, Instagram, Facebook, Whatsapp, and other household names. The Chinese have local substitutes for such giants and are broadly adopted. Without these apps, people there are almost handicapped.

The future of mobile-first
China is one of the countries that is known as a mobile-first country on an important scale. This country has a lot mobile users who are using virtual wallets. From the records of the Ministry of Information and Technology (MIIT) of China, almost 95% of the population of China use mobile devices.

Fastest adoption
The consumers in China are one of the fastest adopting sets in the world when it comes to innovative products and applications. China innovates by focusing on local market needs and through creative adaptation. Various innovative accomplishments of companies in China come from turning an acceptance of local culture into a resourceful adaptation for an innovative consumer need or category. For those who are locals, this frequently comes from the strong perception of an individual in the business who is mostly the founder.

Other countries, or those who want to learn something from China can offer tax incentives to encourage additional large corporations for starting joint ventures along with the entrepreneurial firms every 2 years to make sure that the innovation speed does not hold up or move out of the country.

Business
Entrepreneurial companies which are acquired, at present have the risk of losing their innovative capabilities until they are wrapped up into a larger business where the leading culture might be opposed to more self-governing thought as well as creativity. The learners should follow such companies for their growth and development. One should take long-term views just like what Chinese see for their country and should set objectives and goals that may take several sacrifices and decades; also, keep to them and carry them without splitting and changing every few years.
The Chinese do a lot of background work before making any decision. The specific area where an investment is being measured is visited by the research managers who prepare complete reports for the decision-makers.

In this country, the approval process can be very long and also engage various levels of management; so to get started takes a while. Once it is started, they move at a speed that is far faster than other countries.

Healthcare
The health care system of China includes gratifying physicians for prescribing preventive services. They use trained laypeople as caretakers to the rural areas health care system. The physicians communicate with health policy decision-makers and to the public regarding the significance of including nurses in health

policy decisions and improving the work conditions, staffing, and professional status.

With the improvement in the medical sector of the country and execution of suitable medical and insurance policies, China, however, have achieved what was termed as unattainable by the western powers. The country is on its way to total removal of malaria by the year 2020. So, learning from its unprecedented successes will be extremely valuable to the developing countries facing challenges, as the world is moving towards the achievement of the goals of Sustainable Development.

Education
Education is one of the most vital bases that any country can invest in. Instead of having a child desire to become stars of reality television, it will be better to encourage them to exposure to productive and high-value professions. With the change in attitude of the public toward teachers and holding them in higher esteem, the education system can be developed.

Confucian values and work ethic
China introduced work ethic and Confucian values into their everyday lives. There, the Òme firstÓ orientation is not used. So, just like China, instead of pursuing instant gratification, Confucian values should be preferred or introduced to promote long-term orientation, mutual respect, and reciprocity.

Encouragement of capitalism
The investment in soft and hard infrastructure like

education and smart grid results in the creation of millions of jobs and real wealth in China. This enables large sections of the population to raise themselves into the middle class. Other countries too can have such results by encouraging capitalism in the real economy as a replacement for the financial markets. Support for technology entrepreneurs.

China provides great support to their technology entrepreneurs which facilitate them to focus on filing patents worldwide and also in developing new inventions without any worry of making a living. With support to technology entrepreneurs, other countries can also provide business advice, incubator space, funds for social and financial support of the families of entrepreneurs.

Testing new policies

By testing new policies locally earlier than implementing them countrywide, can facilitate a country to get rid of the problems before it is too late. The government of a country can put forward incentives to states for overseeing their effectiveness and trying out diverse economic programs.

CHAPTER 2 .

ABOUT PROTEINS

The relationship between nutrition and disease is also revealed by Dr. T. Colin Campbell, in this book. He found that a whole-foods diet, which is plant-based cannot only lower the risk for certain diseases,, but can also reverse their evolution.

About 50 years were spent by Dr. Campbell in researching the connection between diet and cancer. The main purpose behind this was to show people how cancer prevention starts with what we put on our plates, and what we do not. According to his book , higher intake of protein is not only unnecessary, but is also a massive problem when it comes to improving cancer risks. Even after getting criticism from the entire food industry and the medical world, he has been a long-time believer that a diet that is high in animal protein intake is a chief cause of cancer.

Research: - From his research, dairy and milk have exclusively been linked to increased risk of cancer. So one of the best things a person can do is giving up dairy in order to decrease their risks of building up cancer cell or cancer. It is found by the researchers in the study that those examined animals who ate a diet that includes 20 percent protein had the highest tumor growth rate, while on the other hand, animals who ate a diet made up of five percent protein had completely no tumor growth. This was done up to three weeks and then the researchers removed the protein from the diet of those animals that had 20 percent protein and the result was that the growth of their tumor completely stopped. This showed that animal protein adds to cancer while plant-based proteins do not. As a result, it was concluded by Dr. Campbell that improved protein consumption is like turning on the switch of cancer, whereas eating least amounts is likened to a switch off.

As we stated before,The China Study states that one should follow a plant-based diet. The plant-based diet, which includes vegetables, leafy greens, nuts, beans, grains, legumes, etc. at each meal, will supply ample of protein, along with nutritious, plant-based nutrients. The China Study also states that the main dissimilarity with plant and animal proteins is their amino acid profiles. Those profiles direct the rates at which the immersed amino acids are set to use within the body. Animal proteins have an advanced concentration of sulphur which contains amino acids that further metabolizes to acid-generating metabolites; thus, a lower physiological pH to some extent must be corrected and barriers like calcium are used to calm the adverse acid effectsÐto the drawbacks of the host. According to The China Study research, the normal adjustment of protein intake was proficient in influencing the capability of a chemical carcinogenÕs capability in the extreme promotion of cancer. The dietary protein trumped a highly strong carcinogen in a species that was extremely sensitive to the carcinogen.

Cholesterol: - The 20-year China Study resulted that the consumption of animal-based foods in high amount is linked with more chronic disease, whereas those intakes primarily a diet which is plant-based were the healthiest. The China Study states that the key of a nutritional dietary overhaul is avoiding dairy, meat and processed foods. A heavy amount of cholesterol and saturated fat is included by animal protein, together with fish, which can put a person at risk for heart disease. The cholesterol is raised by the saturated fats which after a while attack the arteries that further results to strokes and heart attacks. Fish is known for a long time as a good source of omega-3 fatty acids on the other hand 15-30% of it is saturated fat.

Dr. Campbell's recommendation is that one should get protein from vegetables like broccoli (contains 30% protein and high amount absorbable calcium) and beans, like kidney beans, black beans, and pinto beans as they contain a soluble fiber that is helpful in lowering cholesterol. For a good source of protein, we can add whole grains like millet, amaranth, quinoa and nuts like almonds, pistachios, and walnuts as they are all high in protein.

Dr. Campbell links breast cancer to the long-term contact to higher concentrations of the female hormones, which are associated with premature menarche, a high concentration of blood cholesterol, late menopause, and all of these risk factors are linked to a diet high in animal protein and growth.

Kidney stones: - The China Study conclude that the lower the percentage of the animal-based foods that are consumed, the superior the health benefits will be even when that percentage reduces from 10% to 0% of calories. The consumption of animal protein relates to the risk factors for kidney stone formation. The Study state that improved levels of oxalate, as well as calcium in the blood, can result in kidney stones.

Bones: - As per Dr. Campbell, osteoporosis is correlated to the consumption of animal protein based on the reason that animal protein increases the acidity of tissues and blood. To neutralize this acid, calcium is dragged further from the bones, which not only weakens them, but also puts them at higher risk for fracture.

Dr. Campbell and his team state that we do need protein. The Physicians Committee for Responsible Medicine and Center for Disease Control both agree with them to the statement that we are getting ample of protein plus, in our society, the protein deficiency is not a problem particularly in relationship to the problem of cancer we have. They advised that using the RDA (Recommended Dietary Allowance) protein formula, the body weight of an average adult is 0.8 grams per kilogram. They believe that diet can be used to prevent and reverse cancer just the way it reverses and prevents heart disease. A diet which includes high amounts of animal protein not only just increases the quantity of carcinogens leaving in the cells, but also, boosts the enzyme mixed function oxidase (MFO) that results in improved carcinogenic activity.

CHAPTER 3.

HOW TO FIGHT CANCER

There is no doubt in saying that The China Study has taken the country by storm. Nowadays each person is conscious of their health. After the entry of The China Study, numerous people are taking higher control of their health by turning away from traditional meat diets to adopting healthier, plant-based diets.

Through Dr. Campbell, a direct and influential correlation between cancer and animal protein has been made through several experimental, epidemiological evidence, study designs and observation of real life conditions with rational biological description. His book contains thorough accounts of his experiments on laboratory rats where he explained how it was possible to control the growth of cancer on as well as off by just altering the quantity of animal protein that was there in the diet.

He says that every individual has cancer cells at several times in their lives, which sometimes pop up in the bodies. However, what supplies cancer and fortifies it is animal protein. As animal protein adjusts the combination of hormones, it furthermore modifies essential enzyme activities. It causes proliferation of cell, inflammation and creates an acidic atmosphere in the body which then creates a perfect setting for cancer to increase.

While on the other hand, a diet that includes whole plant foods like whole grains, vegetables, beans, and fruits, decreases the risk of various cancers. With such a diet, we get the antioxidants inbuilt in fruits and vegetables that are crucial to defuse cancer causing radicals in the body as well as fiber that acts like a scrub brush going through your body. A plant-based diet is plenty rich in amino acids for the needs of protein. It is a protective diet that is low in saturated fats and high in antioxidants, minerals vitamins, and fiber.

The cells of cancer, which are initiated are not measured to be reversible. Those that develop through the promotion stage are generally measured to be reversible. This stage responds to the nutritional factors. The animal based proteins promote the growth of cancer while the plant-based proteins reverse the promotion stage and react to the nutritional factors. This is a proven observation as cancer proceeds forward or else backward as a role of the stability to promote and anti- promote features found in the diet; therefore, the consumption of anti-promoting plant-based foods help to keep cancer from going forward and possibly even reverse the growth.

The Three Changes
There are particular actions which we need to take today in order to put ourselves on the path to better health as well as superior protection against cancer.

Weigh Less:
Apart from starting a plant-based diet, we should also quit smoking, as well as eating of junk foods. Being less heavy is one vital thing we can do to protect ourselves against various cancers. The plant-based diet will not only provide sufficient nutrients and protein but will also help in losing weight and keeping us fit and healthy.

Eat Smart:
According to health experts, plant-based diet is the healthiest diet. Avoiding alcoholic drinks and animal-based diet or preferring it least like limiting the quantity of cooked red meat to less than 18 ounces per week and staying away from processed meat facilitates in lowering risk for colorectal cancer.

More Movement:
With proper physical activities, we can protect ourselves against cancer directly. The taking of plant-based diet helps in maintaining the body nutrients and protein level. The proper movement of the body by doing physical activities help in removing excess fat. Physical activities regulate hormones that can otherwise encourage the growth of cancer.

On the other hand, we can also limit the consumption of sugary drinks and energy-dense foods. Eat mostly plant-based diet like foods of plant origin, such as fruits, vegetables, legumes and whole grains. Diets high in calcium and dairy products enhance the risk of prostate cancer. Poultry products and fish should not be less taken as they increase the risk of several specific cancers.

In some older studies, it is suggested that the growth of vegetarian children is slower than that of omnivorous. Such children grow slowly at first, but they catch up later. Final heights and weights for vegan children are compared to those of meat-eating children. This is because they get fewer growth-stimulating hormones from their diet; however, it also means a decreased risk of cancer. When a good diet is coupled with other health-promoting activities such as good water, adequate fresh air, exercise, sleep, and sunlight, the benefits will be enormous.

When meat is cooked at high temperatures through pan frying, grilling, or barbecuing potential carcinogenic compounds, heterocyclic amines (HCAs), are formed.These compounds have been strongly linked with increased risk of cancer in several instances.

Dr. Campbell and his team found that a group of diseases, particular cancers of the lung, colon, breast, leukemia, brain, cardiovascular disease, and diabetes were all linked with diets of nutritional excesses. This means a diet that was related to higher level blood urea nitrogen and that of blood cholesterol. These risk pointers were connected directly to the intake of meat, milk, dietary fat, eggs and animal protein plus, inversely linked with legumes and dietary fiber. The mortality of breast cancer is increased with the growing blood cholesterol levels and dietary fat concentration. Higher blood levels, beta-carotene, vitamin C and antioxidants made available by a plant-based diet, were related to lower rates of numerous cancers.

The hypothesis pointed out by The China Study showed that plant-based dietary patterns are high cancer protective than the other standard Western dietary patterns. One of their research also concluded that those animals who ate a diet which consists of 20 percent protein had the maximum tumor growth rate, while, those who ate a diet made up of five percent protein had completely no tumor growth. The rise in consumption of protein turns on the switch of various cancers, whereas eating least amounts result to a switch off. So it's all about the diet of an individual. To stay healthy and live a long life, just go on a plant-based diet.

CHAPTER 4.

OUR HEART

Heart disease is nowadays the number one health problem in almost each country. It is also considered as the leading cause of death. Most heart disease is diet-related and is caused by diets high in animal products.

A vast survey of diet and rates of death from cancer is illustrated by The China Study in more than 2,400 Chinese counties to explore its importance and implications for health and nutrition. The major changes in Chinese society which include a vivid shift from a traditional to a western diet and rapid urbanization, industrialization and lifestyle have contributed to the rise in cardiovascular diseases, like heart attack and stroke. Such changes have been attended by distinct increases in obesity, type 2 diabetes and high cholesterol among the Chinese population.

About 26% of Americans die because of CVD (cardiovascular disease). Each day, about 2,400 people die of it. There is a direct link between a high intake of animal protein and heart disease, high blood pressure, numerous cancers, kidney disease, kidney stones and osteoporosis. The known factors that initiate high blood cholesterol are:-

> Consumption of less plant protein
> Consumption of more animal protein
> Consumption of more saturated animal fat
> Consumption of more cholesterol (present only in animal fat)

The reduction in intake of animal protein and increasing the intake of plant protein is highly important to reduce blood cholesterol. Decreasing animal protein will reduce the saturated animal fat and dietary cholesterol automatically. A vegetarian diet is linked with a less risk of developing heart diseases. Because of high saturated fat content, excess animal protein can raise the risk for heart disease. The animal protein also tends to be advanced in sulfur including amino acids like methionine, which is metabolized to homocysteine; which, in case an individual is not attaining sufficient B12, B6 and folic acid, in their diet, could lead to building up to higher than normal levels.

It is proven in studies that the more plant-based diet, the less the cardiovascular disease death rate, will be. Dietary cholesterol and saturated fat raise the cholesterol of blood. The plant-based diet contains zero cholesterol and in numerous ways, facilitate to reduce the amount of cholesterol made by an individual body. The body is protected by the plants as various plants contain both a large variety of as well as a large concentration of antioxidants which helps to protect the body from harm caused as a result of free radicals. The western diseases are linked to the growth, which is related to the improved risk of initiation, endorsement, and succession of disease plus, that growth is related to a diet which is high in animal protein. The intake of animal protein raises the acidity of tissues and blood; moreover, that also neutralizes this acid and calcium is dragged from the bones.

The lifestyle factors and eating habits play a major role in shaping the risk of heart disease. They may prevent or even overturn this condition. Atherosclerosis is a form of heart disease, in which cholesterol plaques and other substances like small tumors form in the walls of the artery and ultimately restrict the flow of blood. This tense circulation shows the way to less oxygen for the heart muscle, which further results in chest pain during excitement or exercise. The heart muscle is also stressed to the point of failure, which happens during a heart attack. When cholesterol moves into the bloodstream, it is filled into LDL (low-density lipoproteins), also known as the bad cholesterol. Though low-density lipoproteins are essential in limited quantities, a high low-density lipoprotein cholesterol level can significantly raise the risk of a heart attack.

As plenty of cholesterol is made by our bodies for our needs, so there is no necessity to add any in our diet.

In all animal foods like poultry, chicken, red meat, milk, eggs, fish, yogurt, cheese, etc., cholesterol is found. Therefore, for this reason, each animal product should be avoided. On the other side, no plant foods contain cholesterol, as they do not have a liver to produce it. Each 100 mg of cholesterol in daily diet adds about five points to the cholesterol level. Practically 100 mg of cholesterol is included in 4 ounces of chicken or beef and three cups of milk, and half an egg. It is easy to reduce the cholesterol levels noticeably by changing the foods we eat.

Keeping the intake of total fat low, is an essential way to lessen cholesterol and decrease the risk of chronic diseases. For every 1 percent, we can reduce the cholesterol level along with the risk of heart disease by 2 percent. All fried foods and animal products, together with dairy products and meat, are all loaded with fat. Each 10 grams of fiber per day decreases the risk of dying by 10 percent. All fruits and vegetables like beans, barley, Oats, are good sources of soluble fiber. The absorption of some food components like cholesterol is slowed down by soluble fiber. They also decrease the quantity of cholesterol produced by the liver. It is recommended by the experts to take only 20-35 grams of fiber per day. The intake of plant based diet help to consume more fiber from foods which include peas, dried beans, whole grains, cereals, and fruits. The intake of more nuts and fish is associated with considerably lower risk. The individual served with nuts per day is linked with about 30 percent lower risk of heart disease as compared to the one served red meat per day.

According to some studies, nuts are one of the healthiest protein choices that one can make for their heart. The options of nuts include almonds, walnuts, peanuts, pecans, and cashews. Similarly, legumes like peas, beans as well as lentils are an additional excellent option, as they contain no cholesterol and considerably a lesser amount of fat.

Heart disease is nowadays the number one health problem in almost each country. It is also considered as the leading cause of death. Most heart disease is diet-related and is caused by diets high in animal products.

A vast survey of diet and rates of death from cancer is illustrated by The China Study in more than 2,400 Chinese counties to explore its importance and implications for health and nutrition. The major changes in Chinese society which include a vivid shift from a traditional to a western diet and rapid urbanization, industrialization and lifestyle have contributed to the rise in cardiovascular diseases, like heart attack and stroke. Such changes have been attended by distinct increases in obesity, type 2 diabetes and high cholesterol among the Chinese population.

About 26% of Americans die because of CVD (cardiovascular disease). Each day, about 2,400 people die of it. There is a direct link between a high intake of animal protein and heart disease, high blood pressure, numerous cancers, kidney disease, kidney stones and osteoporosis. The known factors that initiate high blood cholesterol are:-

- Consumption of less plant protein
- Consumption of more animal protein
- Consumption of more saturated animal fat
- Consumption of more cholesterol (present only in animal fat)

The reduction in intake of animal protein and increasing the intake of plant protein is highly important to reduce blood cholesterol. Decreasing animal protein will reduce the saturated animal fat and dietary cholesterol automatically. A vegetarian diet is linked with a less risk of developing heart diseases. Because of high saturated fat content, excess animal protein can raise the risk for heart disease. The animal protein also tends to be advanced in sulfur including amino acids like methionine, which is metabolized to homocysteine; which, in case an individual is not attaining sufficient B12, B6 and folic acid, in their diet, could lead to building up to higher than normal levels.

It is proven in studies that the more plant-based diet, the less the cardiovascular disease death rate, will be. Dietary cholesterol and saturated fat raise the cholesterol of blood. The plant-based diet contains zero cholesterol and in numerous ways, facilitate to reduce the amount of cholesterol made by an individual body. The body is protected by the plants as various plants contain both a large variety of as well as a large concentration of antioxidants which helps to protect the body from harm caused as a result of free radicals. The western diseases are linked to the growth, which is related to the improved risk of initiation, endorsement and succession of disease plus, that growth is related to a diet which is high in animal protein. The intake of animal protein raises the acidity of tissues and blood; moreover, that also neutralizes this acid and calcium is dragged from the bones.

The lifestyle factors and eating habits play a major role in shaping the risk of heart disease. They may prevent or even overturn this condition. Atherosclerosis is a form of heart disease, in which cholesterol plaques and other substances like small tumors form in the walls of the artery and ultimately restrict the flow of blood. This tense circulation shows the way to less oxygen for the heart muscle, which further results in chest pain during excitement or exercise. The heart muscle is also stressed to the point of failure, which happens during a heart attack. When cholesterol moves into the bloodstream, it is filled into LDL (low-density lipoproteins), also known as the bad cholesterol. Though low-density lipoproteins are essential in limited quantities, a high low-density lipoprotein cholesterol level can significantly raise the risk of a heart attack.

As plenty of cholesterol is made by our bodies for our needs, so there is no necessity to add any in our diet. In all animal foods like poultry, chicken, red meat, milk, eggs, fish, yogurt, cheese, etc., cholesterol is found. Therefore, for this reason, each animal product should be avoided. On the other side, no plant foods contain cholesterol, as they do not have a liver to produce it. Each 100 mg of cholesterol in daily diet adds about five points to the cholesterol level. Practically 100 mg of cholesterol is included in 4 ounces of chicken or beef and three cups of milk, and half an egg. It is easy to reduce the cholesterol levels noticeably by changing the foods we eat.

Keeping the intake of total fat low, is an essential way to lessen cholesterol and decrease the risk of chronic diseases. For every 1 percent, we can reduce the cholesterol level along with the risk of heart disease by 2 percent. All fried foods and animal products, together with dairy products and meat, are all loaded with fat. Each 10 grams of fiber per day decreases the risk of dying by 10 percent. All fruits and vegetables like beans, barley, Oats, are good sources of soluble fiber. The absorption of some food components like cholesterol is slowed down by soluble fiber. They also decrease the quantity of cholesterol produced by the liver. It is recommended by the experts to take only 20-35 grams of fiber per day. The intake of plant based diet help to consume more fiber from foods which include peas, dried beans, whole grains, cereals, and fruits. The intake of more nuts and fish is associated with considerably lower risk. The individual served with nuts per day is linked with about 30 percent lower risk of heart disease as compared to the one served red meat per day.

According to some studies, nuts are one of the healthiest protein choices that one can make for their heart. The options of nuts include almonds, walnuts, peanuts, pecans, and cashews. Similarly, legumes like peas, beans as well as lentils are an additional excellent option, as they contain no cholesterol and considerably a lesser amount of fat.

CHAPTER 5.

TALKING ABOUT DIABETES

Diabetes is a serious disease, which occurs when sugar accumulates in the blood, and insulin does not work accurately, resulting in numerous problems ranging from vision loss to high blood pressure. Animal based diet is associated with high diabetes risk as they include high protein. The consumption of energy from animal protein at the outflow of energy from either fat or carbohydrates may likewise increase the risk of diabetes.

Individuals who eat protein in high amount, particularly from animal sources, are highly probable to be diagnosed with type 2 diabetes. By animal protein diets an improved sensitivity of insulin is experienced, while those who ate plant-based diet saw a development in their kidney function. A Large quantity of animal protein comes from processed meat and red meat, which have constantly been linked to increased risk of diabetes. Those people who are sensitive to insulin need less amount of insulin to keep their glucose normal; while on the other side those who are resistant to insulin need extra insulin to keep the levels in check.

In The China Study, a great description of diabetes is given by Dr. Campbell which, almost each case of diabetes is either Type 1 or Type 2. The Type 1 diabetes is developed in adolescents and children; so, this is occasionally known as juvenile-onset diabetes, which accounts for 5-10% of all diabetes. Conversely, Type 2 has accounted for 90-95% of each case and occur mostly in adults from age 40 and up, and because of this it is also called adult-onset diabetes. Both Type 1 and Type 2 diabetes have an issue with glucose. When we eat food and it gets digested, glucose is released and then it enters the blood, and so in the pancreas, insulin is produced to transport it all over the body. This procedure breaks down in diabetes. A sufficient amount of insulin cannot be produced by people with Type 1 diabetes because due to autoimmune disease, their pancreas does not function. People with Type 2 diabetics are able to make insulin although, the body does not pay attention to it so, and it does not work. In both Type 1 and Type 2, the outcome is that the glucose is not circulated and increases to risky levels in the blood. When, the glucose leak over into the urine, diabetes is diagnosed. All the sugar in the blood causes various serious complications.

According to Dr. Campbell's research, the rate of Type 2 diabetes has tripled in 25 years, in Japanese children because of increased consumption of animal based diet. The studies show that whole, high-fiber, plant-based diets protect a person against diabetes, while high-protein, high fat, animal-based diets promote diabetes.

Those who take plant-based diets that are, vegetables, beans, and rice, were less likely to develop diabetes as compared to those people whose diets are animal based. The studies recommended that animal-based diets, fatty diets make the body to be more resistant to the actions of insulin. While on other hand adopting a low-fat, plant-based diet does certainly improve the sensitivity of insulin and help out to reduce cholesterol and blood sugar and weight loss.

The plant-based diet is very low in saturated fat and is the kind of fat that is mostly found especially in dairy products, junk food, and meats. So, to effectively cut fat, we will want to do the following:

One is to avoid products that are animal-derived. Unsurprisingly, this will eliminate all animal fats and will eliminate the animal protein. Animal proteins speed up kidney damage in individuals who have already lost a few kidney function. They also increase the loss of calcium from the individual body and the risk of osteoporosis. While the plant sources of protein never create such problems.

Secondly, avoid junk food and additional vegetable oils. While oils are mostly considered as healthier than animal fats, they are also very high in calories, however. So, for the healthiest diet, one will have to keep the oils to a minimum. Just go with the plant based diet. The most significant finding of The China Study was that the more animal protein in an individual's diet like poultry, meat, fish, dairy, and eggs, the higher will be the risk of stroke, heart disease, diabetes, cancer and obesity that such individual would have.

Sufficient amount of dietary protein intake in type 2 diabetes is of particular importance as proteins are somewhat neutral in connection with lipid metabolism and glucose, and they safeguard the mass of muscle and bone, which possibly decrease in matters with diabetes which is poorly controlled.

A late postprandial increase in the glucose levels of blood is exerted in ingestion of diabetes type 1 dietary protein because of the stimulation of protein, so as to encourage pancreatic glucagon emission. The study also verified the bringing of animal protein into the data set. The study cleared that, High carbs countries had a large amount of lower diabetes rates, and the one with the uppermost diabetes rate, had a classic western diet, which is high in animal fat, calories, total fat and animal protein. Those who had lower diabetes rates mostly ate a plant-based diet or a lot of rice. It was also found that diabetes was highly related to excess cholesterol and weight.

The China Study evaluated urine tests, blood tests, health histories, dietary questionnaires, the direct size of diet and health histories by looking into 65 different regions and the diet and health of about 6500 people. The result of the research ended up with over 8000 numerically important relations between diet, lifestyle, and disease.

It was concluded that diabetes is a disease, which can be managed through plant-based diet, insulin medication suitable management and physical activities. A regular intake of plant-based diet could lead to uptake of healthy glucose. Eating plant-based foods that take longer to reach the bloodstream and digest slowly, source insulin to release gradually and help the body in maintaining the perfect level of glucose.

CHAPTER 6.

THE CHINA STUDY AND OBESITY

There is no doubt in saying that the risks of the number of chronic diseases increase with the obesity. Obesity increases the chances of hypertension, dyslipidemia, cardiovascular disease, certain types of cancer and diabetes. It is a complex crisis that needs action at various levels, including government, institutional, non-government organizations and significantly industry.

The China Study by Dr. Campbell and his team has found that consumption of meat is linked to obesity. The China Study found that eating meat is a serious concern for the modern diet and health of humans, as the protein directly contributes to the universal obesity crisis. This is the basis that meat protein takes much more time than fats and carbohydrates. It is digested later and makes all the energy gained from protein an excess, which is then transformed and stored in the body as fat.

The intake of animal based diet increases the insulin whose secretion works in a variety of ways to slow down the oxidation of fat and promote fat storage. The dietary protein powers body weight by disturbing four targets for weight regulation of body which are body composition, thermogenesis, satiety, and energy efficiency.

According to the experts, studies show that intake of plant protein has a higher power to lesser levels of cholesterol than reducing the intake of fat or cholesterol. During the research of The China Study, the death rate from the coronary heart disease was about seventeen times superior among American men than the rural Chinese men. They cleared that a protein diet can cause little shifts in the metabolism of calorie that cause big shifts in body weight. The results of the study showed that all those individuals who had the highest consumption of meat or animal products were also reported with the highest rates of obesity. The consumption of meat is as similar to sugar.

The China Study present physicians an update regarding life-saving nutritional information with the help of plant-based diets. The study examines the relationship between illnesses such as diabetes, obesity, cancers of the breast, large intestine, prostate, autoimmune disease, osteoporosis, macular degeneration and degenerative brain disease and the consumption of animal products. This is because the proteins in animal product or meat are mostly digested at a slower rate as compared to fats and carbohydrates. A caloric surplus can be created by the meat sources in the meals.

The China Study emphasizes that the rates of obesity are as a result of a dynamic contact of the sources and types of food we eat. The excess consumption of meat by the individuals is likely to cause obesity because of excess sugar consumption. Fruits, beans, and vegetables are the plant based diets which are high in fiber and is not immersed into the bloodstream. Because of this reason, some of the weight of these plant-based foods does not convert into calories intake. According to Dr. Campbell, the average calorie intake per kilogram of body weight as much higher among the Chinese that is less active than among the average Americans; so, body weight was much lower. The consumption of diets high in fat and protein transfers the calories which are absent to body heat and stored as body fat.

A diet can cause small shifts in calorie metabolism which further causes great shifts in body weight. Low-fat diet help to prevent obesity and permit people to attain their full development potential. The studies show that plant-based foods, whole, high-fiber, protect against high-fat, diabetes and high-protein while the animal based foods promote diabetes. The increase in expenditure of energy is led by synthesis of protein, gluconeogenesis, and urea. It is an effect which is advanced with animal-based diets as their protein contain a great amount of important amino acids. Consumption of advanced amounts of protein throughout dietary treatment of obesity results in better weight loss as compared with lower amounts of protein in nutritional studies lasting up to a year.

Plant based diet helps a person to lose weight easily. During weight loss as well as reduced caloric intake, a comparatively improved protein content of the diet, maintain improved calcium balance and fat-free mass which results in bone mineral content preservation.

The considerable natural weight loss regularly seen with regimens of very-low-fat dietary may result in a reduced rate of fat ingestion along with an enhanced insulin sensitivity of skeletal muscle that regulates down the insulin discharge.

The dietary protein provokes small insulin release by itself and can clearly potentiate the reaction of insulin to consume carbohydrate. In western meals, the secretion of postprandial insulin may be reduced by avoiding animal-based diets. This is because western meals are mostly starchy foods as well as animal-based diet; so they should be avoided.

Healthy eating may be achieved with the intake of a plant-based diet. The plant-based diet is a regimen that supports plant-based foods, and it is whole and put off eggs, dairy products, meats as well as all processed and refined foods. The research in The China Study also shows that the plant-based diets are not only just cost-effective but are also low-risk interventions that have the power to lower body mass index, control blood pressure, cholesterol levels and HbA1C. They also have the power to reduce a variety of medications required to lower ischemic heart disease mortality rates and treat chronic diseases.

It was found that vegetarian populations contain lower rates of high blood pressure, heart disease, obesity and diabetes. In addition, weight loss in such population is not dependent on exercise, as it occurs at a rate of about 1 pound per week. A vegan diet resulted in burning calories in large amount after meals, as compared to those who intake animal based diet, which may cause the least amount of calories to be burned.

CHAPTER 7.

THE MOST DANGEROUS CANCERS: BREAST, PROSTATE, COLON & RECTAL

The China Study includes a great research of numerous years done with an objective to know the relation between intake of animal products, plant products, protein, plus, meat and the risk of various cancers like breast, prostate, colon and rectal. With his book, Dr. Campbell has taken the countries by storm, and as a result, each person has now been conscious of health.

The China Study explained how the consumption of meat based products gives rise to health diseases. It showed that countries with an advanced intake of fat, chiefly fat from animal-based diet or products, like dairy and meat products, have an advanced incidence of breast cancer. In Japan, the traditional diet is very less in fat, particularly animal fat as compared to the typical western diet and it was recorded in the study that the breast cancer rates are low.

Animal products mentioned in The China Study included various foods like meat and meat products along with their categories, shellfish, fish and dairy products like yogurt, milk, cheese, and eggs. The study concluded that the consumption of all such high-fat foods causes a person's body, especially women, to make estrogens in high amount, which further gives rise to the growth of cancer cell in the breast as well as other organs that are highly sensitive to an individual's sex hormone. The China Study suggests that the avoidance of fatty foods is of great benefits to an individual throughout life. This avoidance helps in decreasing the risk of cancer due to hormones and other various reasons.

When the amount of fat is reduced by the diet, their levels of estrogen were held at a safer and lower level in the next several years. The increase in intake of fruits, vegetables, beans, grains, and reduction in animal-based foods, the quantity of estradiol in the blood dropped to a great level as compared to those who did not alter their diets.

When the scientists researched the links between cancer and diet, it was found that people who avoided meat were much less likely to develop the disease. The animal products like meat contain saturated fat, animal protein in much amount and, in a few cases, carcinogenic compounds like PAH (polycyclic aromatic hydrocarbons) and HCA (heterocyclic amines) which are formed throughout the cooking or processing of meat. When meat is cooked at high temperatures, the HCAs and PAHs, formed at the time of the burning of organic substances, are known to enhance the risk of cancer. The high-fat content of animal based products and meat raises the production of the hormone which raises the risk of hormone-related cancers like breast as well as prostate cancer.

The study cleared that animal based diet has numerous disadvantages while a plant-based diet has numerous advantages. It is a fact that plant-based diets like vegetables include plant estrogens (phytoestrogens) which help the body to normalize the amount of testosterone to estrogen. The animal based diet just raise them and increase the chances of cancer, while plant-based diet decreases this risk to a great level.

With the globalization of habits of Western eating, the risk of Prostate cancer appears to be growing worldwide. Cancer is linked to higher dairy intake and meat and diets low in fiber and rich in processed foods along with processed meat, refined grains, red meat, and fast foods. On the other hand, a plant-based or low–fat, vegetarian diet facilitates to stop prostate cancer and play an important role in its treatment.

The China Study suggests that a vegetarian or plant-based diet is highly helpful in the treatment, prevention as well as reversal of cancer. An evident rise in the relative risk of breast cancer is found in the study with the increase in consumption of meat.

The considerably lower pH in the colon because of a plant-based diet facilitates to lower the threat of colon cancer. The plant-based foods like beans, broccoli, and fruits like berries, strawberries, and nuts, sweet potatoes are all protective foods that play a vital role in preventing colon cancer. There is a starch known as resistant starch, which has its origin from plant-based foods such as raw oatmeal, cooked peas, beans, lentils. They have the ability to block the accumulation of highly harmful effects of metabolism of animal protein in the colon. A large amount of iron in the body, particularly the type that comes from animal based foods or meat increases the risk of colon cancer. The consumption of protein found in animal foods is connected with a hormone called IGF-1, which makes an increase in a cancer-promoting growth. However, the power of plant-based diet and lifestyle changes helps to improve cancer survival.

The China Study has shown that the intake of dairy products and dietary fat raises the risk of prostate cancer, whereas the compounds found in plant foods like soy, tomatoes and various vegetables protect against the disease. Similarly, the calcium from dairy products was linked to prostate cancer risk. The results support the research data that a high consumption of calcium or protein from dairy products raises the risk of prostate cancer.

The consumption of cruciferous vegetables like cabbage, broccoli, Brussels sprouts, and cauliflower, is also related to reduce risk of prostate cancer. The China Study cleared the reason behind this, and it is because these foods can encourage phase II detoxification enzymes along with apoptosis and cell–cycle arrest in prostate cancer cells. So, the perfect healthy diet is not an animal-based diet, but, the plant-based diet. T. Colin Campbell recommends eating daily a plant-based diet to stay away from such dangerous diseases and live a healthy and fit life. With this, we can also say that the data of The China Study is not only interesting but is also highly helpful in Perfect Health Diet.

CHAPTER8.

THE CHINA STUDY AND

AUTOIMMUNE DISEASES

The China Study book also helps people in numerous ways by bringing to light the relationship between plant-based diets, animal-based diets, and human health. The China Study also stated that a plant-based diet was key to staying free from autoimmune diseases.

Plant-based diets have the ability to successfully treat various autoimmune diseases like rheumatoid arthritis, multiple sclerosis, Lichen planus, Crohn's disease and some types of cancer, which may contain an autoimmune component.

For the growth of autoimmune diseases, systemic inflammation may pay a regular contribution. When the tissues of the body are attacked by its own immune system, autoimmune disease (AD) takes place. The immune system is a multipart set in the body that is designed to destroy and seek the invaders of the body, together with the infectious agents. Individuals with autoimmune diseases commonly have unusual antibodies moving in their blood that destroy the tissues of their own body.

With the intake of animal-based diet like meat, a low-grade inflammation is experienced by the body because of the appearance of bacterial endotoxins within the bloodstream. Such diet includes arachidonic acid, which may directly make the immune system active and further promote inflammation. The highly concentrated ingested animal hormones are found in low-fat dairy, which may also keep hold of some physiological function and potentially encourage the pathological activation of immune.

The consumption of meat also causes rheumatoid arthritis. This happens with meat intake to antibody production in opposition to Proteus mirabilis bacteria, which cross-react in the end with the proteins in joint tissue. Whereas, the consumption of a plant-based diet does not give such results. They don't generate similar phenomena, as plant based diets are simply too different from our own. Plants are highly rich in potassium which can encourage the creation of natural steroids that helps to hold back inflammatory processes. Animal-based diets also contain live contaminating bacteria which are known to cause autoimmune diseases directly.

Autoimmune diseases like rheumatoid arthritis (RA), psoriasis (Ps) multiple sclerosis (MS), inflammatory bowel disease (IBD) and type 1 diabetes (T1D) are a heterogeneous group of diseases by which common characteristics along with the participation of multifactorial etiologies, a course of chronic clinical that regularly requires lifelong disease management and a mediated autoimmune pathology mechanisms of T cell is shared. With the growth of inflammatory autoimmune diseases, genetic factors is undoubtedly affected. However, for most of the diseases within the monozygotic twins, environmental factors play a relatively low concordance rate as important triggers of disease.

According to Dr. Campbell, in his collection of years of nutritional research, "The China Study," the animal-based proteins (particularly dairy), which is partially digested or undigested have the chances of leaking out from the slightly permeable intestinal wall of an individual into the blood stream. They fuel the development and growth of malignancies as well as cause autoimmune and arthritis flare-ups.

This outflow of protein is actually the foreign protein within the bloodstream. The plant-based diet includes proteins that do not have adverse effects like arthritis, autoimmune responses, and malignancies. Plant based protein is never taken as foreign protein within the bloodstream. The foreign protein linked to the animal based protein is not only just responsible for arthritis and malignancies, but is also responsible for various autoimmune diseases like pernicious diabetes, Cranes Disease, anemia, lupus, MS, arthritis, Gravis, autoimmune disorders related to Kidney, myasthenia gravisHashimoto disease.

The intake of gluten can also cause the condition of the foreign protein. Some individuals are highly allergic to it and several people have gluten sensitivity; however, they are not even aware of it, as the sensitivity of gluten is cleared by some autoimmune diseases, without having any connection to gluten as the cause.

Before the beginning of autoimmune conditions and malignancies, a highly capable immune system is proficient of destroying the most free-radical cells. Moreover, the undigested animal-based proteins are prevented by a highly proficient digestive system along with the gluten from going into the bloodstream. Most people do not have such a digestive system or immune system that is highly efficient, and because of this, they have to face the consequences of the foreign protein in the blood which results from the intake of animal-based proteins and gluten from dairy products like yogurt, milk, cheese, etc. The China Study found that the western diet is also responsible for dysfunctional digestion of the nutrients and poor efficiency of the immune system, as they lack in adequate amounts of live enzymes and antioxidants. Plant-based diets are rich in potassium, which have the ability to stimulate the creation of natural steroids required to hold back the inflammatory processes.

It is revealed by the research of Dr. Campbell, that milk protein which is found in casein, cheese, in milk, yogurt, sour cream and other dairy products is more likely to improve the malignancies metastasizing and speed up the development of arthritis as well as other autoimmune conditions the same as animal based proteins. Animal based diet increases the risk of breast cancer that had metastasized to the bone and lungs.

43

The intake of a 100% plant-based diet keeps a person healthy, fit and away from all such diseases.

There are multiple explanations of how the "western lifestyle" favors the development of autoimmunity. The hypothesis of hygiene states that the western lifestyle and food increase the risk of factors to autoimmune diseases. The regular consumption of fast food and lack of physical activity causes a high chance of obesity, which, in turn, result in cardiovascular and metabolic disease and also constitute as risk factors to the autoimmune diseases.

A plant-based diet, which is rich in enzymes, consist of daily intake of raw fruits and vegetables, which, helps to strengthen the digestive function and immune system. They have a dramatic and positive effect on the general health of an individual and cures autoimmune diseases, cancer, infections and other conditions.

CHAPTER 9.

CONCLUSION

There is no doubt that a poor diet can show the way to numerous chronic diseases together with obesity, cardiovascular disease, and type 2 diabetes. After the entry of The China Study and several research studies done by Dr. T. Colin Campbell and his team, it is clear to each person that eating healthy is highly important. However, it is not so easy to find a diet that is not just nutritious, but, also sustainable.

With the intention of having a healthy diet, a lot of advice and much confusion exist, regarding what a person should and what not eat. The term diet means that a particular diet is prescribed or regulated for precise reasons that are mostly related to health. In The China Study, after wide investigations over numerous it was concluded that a vegetarian, whole food, diet prevents as well as reverses several diseases and have the ability to extend lives, and turn off cancer.

The conclusive evidence is offered by The China Study, that a change of diet can significantly decrease the risks of obesity, heart disease, and diabetes. The China Study conveys a holistic sight of nutrition.

A healthy lifestyle has enormous benefits like to lose weight, prevent and treat diabetes, lower the blood pressure, live a fuller life, more energy, lower the risk of prostate, breast, and various other cancers, look and feel younger, lower the blood cholesterol, alleviate constipation, prevent as well as reverse heart disease, and many more. But to take all such benefits, a proper diet is required. So, The China Study has mentioned some Principles of Food and Health that promote health.

#1 Principle: Nutrition represents the combined activities of countless food substances. The whole is greater than the sum of its parts.

This principle means that if you are struggling in adopting a lifestyle which is plant-based and slips up from time to time, then there is no need to be hard on yourself. Each plant-based diet includes distinctive nutrients which are very important to our body. The foods contain chemicals that engaged in a sequence of reactions that work in performance to generate good health. They are arranged carefully by complex controls within the cells and through the bodies. Our bodies have evolved with this infinitely complex network of reactions in order to derive maximal benefit from whole food, as they appear in nature." Understanding what good nutrition mean is essential to good health. We can live a life which is healthier than the day before, and the overall health is affected by the decisions taken by a majority, not by those in the minority.

#2 Principle: Vitamin supplements are not a panacea for good health.
The China Study bring to light that supplements never lead to a long-lasting health, but can source unexpected side effects. Just by consuming the pills of nutrient, the risks of a Western diet cannot be overcome. The beneficial and constant diet change is delayed by those who rely on supplements. The intake of a diet that gives all the nutritional components in great amount, is a straightforward alternative. With the diet based on whole foods, we can get all the nutrients without any fear of side effects.

#3 Principle: There are virtually no nutrients in animal-based foods that are not better provided by plants.
It is clear by The China Study that, plant-based diet has more minerals, antioxidants, and fiber as compared to the animal-based diets. Various vegetables provide high levels of plant protein. Plant-based foods reverse the symptoms of chronic pain, aging, and also helps in losing weight.

#4 Principle: Genes do not determine disease on their own. Genes function only being activated, or expressed, and nutrition plays a critical role in determining which genes, good and bad, are expressed.

Genes are the code to everything in our bodies, whether it is good or bad. In determining this, nutrition plays an important role. As, it is known to each gardener that, without proper sunshine, water, and nutrient-rich soil, the seeds will not grow up into plants. Similarly, nutrition is the factor that decides the activity of genes. Unless genes have the proper environment, they cannot express.

#5 Principle: Nutrition can substantially control the adverse effects of noxious chemicals.

The China Study says nobody wants to hear that their favorite foods can cause them trouble due to their nutritional content. Whatever we take, is broken down into substances and chemicals by the body, which further have a positive or negative impact. Those who take animal-based foods will later experience more cancer as well as heart disease. Whether the disease will harm or not depends on the nutritional intake.

#6 Principle: The same nutrition that prevents disease in its early stages can also halt or reverse disease in its later stage.

Chronic diseases take some years to develop. They do not take place overnight. It is shown in various research that with the help of good nutrition and a plant-based diet, the diseases can be slowed or even reversed. When we take nutrition from plant-based diets, they will halt or reverse the disease in its later stage.

#7 Principle: Nutrition that is truly beneficial for one chronic disease will support health across the board.

We all know how beneficial a plant-based diet is. But, we should also be aware that plant-based diet taken by us will not promote any other disease while stopping the one at hand. A plant based diet will not only help in losing weight but will also help with symptoms of the diseases and lose pain.

#8 Principle: Good nutrition creates health in all areas of our existence. All parts are interconnected.

Food and nutrition are extremely important to our health; however, mental and emotional health, physical activity, good environment are too essential for us. A healthy diet decreases the chances of facing particular diseases like cancer and develops the capability to enjoy our life to the fullest. A plant-based diet, which is when combined with a good routine of exercise is the easy solution to our daily miseries.

ABOUT THE AUTHOR

Russell Dawson, is a health, diet and food writer, and develops acid alkaline food, Paleo Diet, and low-carb and gluten-free recipes for home cooks. Experience:

Russell has been developing health and education Web sites for over 3 years. He has been focusing on acid-alkaline balance diet, Paleo Diet, and low-carb and low-glycemic eating for more than 3 years -- investigating the emerging science related to low-carb eating, writing articles to help people change their diets, and developing healthy menus and recipes.

OTHERS BOOKS BY RUSSELL DAWSON

To Check Out All My Books, visit my site:
http://www.RussellDawsonBooks.com

21815938R00035

Printed in Great Britain
by Amazon